HOMEMADE SHAMPOO

How to Treat Your Hair with Natural and
Organic Homemade Shampoo and
Make it Shiny & Healthy
(Shampoo Making and Recipes)

By ERIK FISHNER

Table of Contents

Introduction

In our ever-changing world, the need to get back to basics has become a prominent movement over the last decade. The realization of the harm that humans have created on this planet has provoked this movement. Being "green" is no longer a choice, but more of a moral obligation. Ecologically minded people have banned together to come up with positive solutions to perpetuate an earth-conscious mindset. Communities as a whole are becoming more self-sustaining. Within this ecological inspiration, each individual looks at what they can do to contribute. They are finding the best way to initiate Eco mindfulness, is right in their own homes!

The products we use daily for hygiene and beauty, are chemical ridden and costly. There have been studies that define the link between these harmful products to several undesirable results on our health. Their production leads to more waste, harming the environment further. It is for the better of everyone that we stop contributing to the poisoning of the planet, and ourselves.

When we begin our quest for knowledge on how to benefit our family and ourselves with ecologically sound choices, the amount of information can be overwhelming. So, why not start with the basics? We all enjoy looking and feeling our best.

What better way to reflect your healthy, ecological positive lifestyle, than a gorgeous head of hair?

Together, we'll explore alternatives to store bought shampoos. We'll learn to use organic, natural ingredients to achieve hair health and growth. With accessible recipes, you'll be on your way to lovely locks!

Chapter 1: A Hairy Situation - All about Hair

Since early humans, hair has marked what we are. Hair was thought to hold the power of our thoughts. Our hair communicates visual messages. It's an outward expression of our being. Hair reflects our sensuality, our relationship with our body. By looking at another's hair, we assess them; evaluate their position in comparison to our own. Concepts of beauty have a deep connection with the way we ornament our hair. Every year, time and resources are spent for the sole purpose of hair grooming.

Hair's chemistry is unique to each individual, holding the secrets of our DNA. Hair also has information about anything that has ever entered into your blood stream. Our hair is an amazing storage place for our health history. The only thing unidentifiable in hair genetics is the sex of the owner. All our hair structure is the same, no matter whose head it's on.

Hair grows quickly, being one of the fastest growing tissues of the human body. The hair on the human head grows at a rate of 0.3 to 0.5 millimeters daily. Hair is extremely strong, nearly an indestructible part of us. Hair strands can be stretched up to 30% of its own length, when wet. That our hair continues to grow after death, is a well-known myth, but is actually true by technicality. The body begins to lose moisture after death; therefore pulling back, exposing more hair. We measure hair length from where the hair meets the skin to the tip, so technically the hair does "grow". Each strand of hair can bear one hundred grams of weight. For a full head of hair, that's about two tons!

Hair's strength is often compared to that of a copper wire. Each hair contains its own muscle, blood and nerve supply. The lifespan of one single hair is approximately five years. A healthy hair follicle can replace a new strand of hair up to twenty times in an average lifespan. Hair protects us, maintains our body temperature acting as a natural insulator. Due to the fact that our heads have substantially less fat than that of the rest of our bodies, hair provides the extra protective heat layer.

Hair is made up of keratin, the same protein material found in animal hooves, claws, and beaks. All the hair follicles that we will ever have are developed in the womb, at approximately five months of gestation. They slowly decrease as we age. The hair on our heads acts as a natural sponge. Depending on your natural hair color, you can have up to 150,000 strands on your head. Natural blondes have more hair than natural red heads. We shed out hair daily, from forty to one hundred and fifty strands. All our hair structure is the same; it is the follicles that determine straightness or curliness. Hair follicles also determine the thickness and length of your hair.

All your hair is completely dead, except for the part that is still on your scalp. The growing phase of body hair is shorter than the growing phase of the hair on your scalp. That is the reason body hair is generally shorter than the hair that is on your head. Scientific studies have shown that people with higher IQ's have more of the minerals zinc and copper in their hair strands. There are up to fourteen different types of mineral element in your hair, including traces of gold.

Our hair is an extremely interesting subject, and there is a plethora of information available about the subject. The above facts are just a glimpse into the amazing world of hair.

Chapter 2: A Short History of Hair - Myths and Legends

Hair is often the first thing that people notice about us. It is an extremely important factor in determining your attractiveness to another. It is used to express personality, mood, and beliefs. There are so many ways to style, manipulate and color your hair these days. In the days of yore, hair was often seen as a wondrous extension of the head, where the thoughts are formed. Based on these perceptions, many myths, and legends been passed down about our mystical hair. Let's explore some of the most popular ones.

~224 BC

Berenice the second, the Seleucid queen of Egypt, cut her beautiful long hair, offering it in sacrifice to Aphrodite. She did this to ensure the safe return of her husband from the wars in Syria. He did return safely. His wife's hair sacrifice, however, was stolen by a priest of the temple where she had left it. He justified his thievery by stating the sacrifice was to a Greek deity, and not one of their own. This was only because queen Berenice was Seleucid. The court astronomer Konon was called upon to remedy the situation. He quickly stated that the goddess had accepted her offering; put it in the sky, turning it into a cluster of stars that shine in the Galactic North Pole. This solution named the constellation,"Coma Berenices".

~Indo-European

Sif in Nordic myths and legends was a wife of Thor. Her hair cascaded past his feet. One fine day, the tricky god, Loki, cut it all off and ran away with it. Upon discovering her hair cut, Sif wailed in grief. Hearing his wives' crying and suffering, Thor vowed the worst punishment for Loki. Loki, fearful of Thor, sought help from the dwarves. The dwarves wove the hair with gold, making the hair longer than before. Loki brought this to Sif as an apology, and Thor was appeased.

~Medusa

Medusa is not a tale of hair beauty, but one of terror. She was one of the three Gorgon sisters. Being priestess of Athena's temple, Medusa was once a beautiful maiden. Then she was raped by Poseidon, who in his fury transformed her hair into snakes, and disfigured her face so that anyone who looked upon it instantly turned to stone. She was killed by Perseus, by her own reflection in a mirror. Perseus brought her head back as a trophy to Athena, who then used it as a shield.

~Samson

A judge of the ancient Israelites, Samson was said to be similar to the Greek's Hercules, in strength and power. Samson grew up fulfilling an angel's prophecy that he would liberate the Hebrews of the Philistines. Part of his oath was to never cut or shave his hair. His hair was the secret of his strength, and he went on to perform many heroic deeds; much like Hercules. Samson falls in love with a woman, Delilah, who learns of his secret. Delilah proves to be treacherous, in that she was bribed by the Philistines. She betrays Samson and cuts his hair as he sleeps. She delivers Samson's hair to the Philistines. Robbed of his source of strength, Samson becomes enslaved. Samson did not remain enslaved for much time, as his hair quickly grew back. With his hair regrowth, his strength returned. At a gathering in the temple, many Philistines were crushed when Samson pulled two pillars together. He died with the Philistines, but not without his vengeance.

As you've read, there are many interesting myths that surround hair. It is an enormous factor in attractiveness and appeal. As humans, we are drawn to hair that is creatively styled. Hair can help define what you'd like to represent to the world, the image that you'd like to portray.

Many legendary women have had long, beautiful hair. Long hair has been associated with femininity throughout history. Venus uses her long hair to conceal her attributes in the famous painting, "The birth of Venus" by Botticelli. Since long hair often demonstrates good health, it is highly sought after by most women. Also, some men have grown their hair as a display of nonconformity. Many famous men are noted for their hair. The Beatles are a prime example of how much hair affects the way we are perceived. One of the biggest factors that made them stand out beside their obvious musical talent was their shaggy hairstyle.

Whether it is short or long, our interest in hair has a long history.

This history can be further developed by understanding what we put on our hair for the sake of beauty and cleanliness.

Chapter 3: Ecologically Sound Hair - Hair Care Products and Their Toll on You and the Environment

We give a lot of thought into taking care of our hair. From daily shampooing to visits to the hair stylist, we love grooming our hair. When we choose products for our hair, three main things come into play.

Does it smell nice?
Is it cost efficient?
And lastly, will it create an overall improvement in my hair?

Many products out on the market cover these three basics, quite easily. Then they go even further, making outrageous claims. They draw you in with their unique packaging and promises. Big companies are hugely successful, in that hair care product sales range in the billions, yearly. How much is actually true? Can we rely on these big money makers to be concerned about our health? Can we trust them to care for our environment?

Mostly the answer is no. Although most hair care products ingredients are listed on the packaging, they can be confusing if you aren't experienced with chemistry or the periodic table of elements. Habitually, only ten percent of the population *really* reads ingredient labels, and about the same percentage understand them. Why would companies do this? For profit, the companies cannot subsidize Mother Nature, so they sell you an idea about their "natural" product. In general, these mass producers of hair care products don't set out to harm the public, but the cocktail of chemicals they put into their products can have adverse effects on our health.

The main hair care product pertaining to this book is shampoo. Let's check it out. The shampoo comes from the Hindi word "champo", which roughly translates into the massage. The shampoos we know of today, that we use in the western hemisphere, have been in use since approximately the 1930s. Before that, shampoo was derived from the byproducts of boiled down soaps. Much before that, shampoos were more natural, using plant based ingredients. From ancient times to now, shampoo and its ingredients have changed fundamentally.

With these changes, came the commercialization of shampoo. Its mixture of chemicals and the need for packaging harms the world in which we live.

With the onset of the ecological movements in the early 1970s, big time producers have "gone green", and made claims on their products. They proclaim organic ingredients and environmentally sound practices. They claim their packaging is recyclable. Although, in some cases, there may be truth to their claims; unfortunately, their claims are mostly untrue. They are untrue, in the sense that they meet scant federal regulation to be able to advertise their product as "green". They place floral designs on their bottles, along with colors that have been conjured up in marketing studies, to give the consumer a sense of ecological safety.

Yet, these products still contain preservatives, bonding agents, and foaming agents! The omission of some truths by the big corporations is not news. Otherwise, how would they turn over a profit to continue producing? Based on our western notion of cleanliness, and the constant need for it, these companies are laughing all the way to the bank.

Modern shampoos work by the way of surfactants. Surfactants work by lowering the interfacial tension between two liquids or a liquid and a solid. Surfactants can be wetting agents, detergents, foaming agents, and emulsifiers. Shampoo uses a particular type of surfactant, being balanced so as not to strip the hair completely of oil. Surfactants are not the main problem in shampoo, but it depends on what combination is in the product, and with what other chemicals. The most common type of surfactant in common shampoos is anionic surfactants. Anionic surfactants reduce the interfacial surface tension, allowing for sebum removal from the hair shaft. Sebum is natural oil secreted by our hair follicles. Sebum is beneficial for our hairs protection, although it needs to be regulated through washing, stripping it does not lead to healthy hair. When your shampoo foams up, it is nothing but aesthetics, foaminess serves no purpose except to fool us into thinking of cleanliness. By being constantly bombarded with the idea of germs, we easily buy into this foamy lie.

How can we become responsible contributors to our environment and health? By having complete control over what we put on our bodies, and by using ecologically responsible container units for storage. But wait, we don't want to give up shampoo entirely, because it does help our hair to restore itself. The shampoo does have many benefits for our hair health and scalp cleanliness. What we can do, is start with the basics, using natural ingredients that we know come from a natural and organic origin. When we make this change, we change our hair's health. We change our attitude towards harmful chemicals, refusing to buy into commercial shampoo's illusion.

From a basic recipe, you can create shampoo specific for you and your family's needs. In the next chapters, we will investigate how we can successfully maintain a healthy head of hair while demonstrating our concern for the environment.

Chapter 4: Back to Basics - Tools for Making Your Own Shampoo

Shampoo making with natural ingredients will give you the opportunity to learn a new skill. With this new skill, you can mindfully contribute to your hair's health. You will be able to know, very well, every ingredient and its source. Packaging will be selected by you. You will have the ability to choose the most environmental-friendly options. Imagine the delight of those around you, having a custom made shampoo on hand! To begin the process, you will need some tools. These may be easily acquired in your local kitchen shop or online. For liquid shampoo, you can purchase pump bottles. You can also recycle mason jars. For bar shampoo, you may need a wood mold, or you can use deep dish oven pans lined with parchment paper. You will most certainly need essential oils, herbs, and different base oils. Again, all these are easily acquired.

Give yourself the time to make your shampoo. It isn't time-consuming, but taking the time to correctly measure the ingredients is important. Ensure that you have adequate space to accommodate your ingredients and tools. Be patient, it is a learning process. You will soon know exactly what best suits your needs.

The following is a basic list of tools for liquid shampoos*:

- (Organic) castile soap
- Storage bottles - these can be pump, spray or just recycled jars
- Variety of essential oils
- Honey
- Coconut oil
- Olive oil
- Funnel

*These ingredients may vary from recipe to recipe, the only thing that doesn't change is the need for storage.

The following is for bar shampoos*:

- (Organic) pure soap for melting (melt and pour)
- Crock pot or stove top pan used *only* in bar shampoo making
- Microwave
- Soap molds (wood or bread pan with parchment paper)
- Variety of essential oils
- Soap dish for storage

*These ingredients may vary from recipe to recipe, the only thing that doesn't change is the need for pure soap for melting.

The following is for dry shampoos*:

- (Organic) dried roots from local herbalist or market
- Storage containers

- Baking soda

*These ingredients may vary from recipe to recipe, the only thing that doesn't change is the need for storage.

Now that we have the basics covered, let's begin to create our own shampoos.

To decide what type of shampoo you would like to make, consider your habits, and which suits you best. Having one of each type on hand is a wonderful way to be prepared to master skills as a shampoo maker.

Chapter 5: Liquid Shampoo Recipes - Recipes for all Types of Hair

Our first set of liquid shampoo recipes will be for oily hair. Be sure to know very well what type of hair you have, to make the shampoo that will work best for your hair.

Oily hair can be detected by these signs:

- Your hair appears dull
- Your hair gets very greasy soon after washing
- Your hair looks lifeless and limp

Any of these signs, or a combination of them, could mean you have oily hair. To better determine your hair type, consult a professional stylist. Use the following recipes as you would shampoo.

Oil Away Shampoo

You will need:
A large bowl used exclusively for shampoo making
Spoon or spatula to mix
Funnel

Jar for storage

Ingredients:
11 drops of tea tree oil
1 tablespoon of liquid organic castile soap
1 tablespoon of green clay
1 teaspoon of brewed green tea (strong)
How to:
Mix all the ingredients in the bowl until smooth. It will have a muddy consistency. Scoop it into the jar. It can be stored up to three days.

Fresh and Oil Free Shampoo

You will need:
A large bowl used exclusively for shampoo making
Spoon or spatula to mix
Funnel
Jar for storage/bottle

Ingredients:
½ cup of boiled water
2 tablespoons of freshly chopped mint (organic)
1 tablespoon of fresh rosemary (organic)
¼ cup of organic castile soap

How to:

Pour the water into the bowl. Mix in the rosemary and mint. Add the castile soap. Allow the mixture to steep for an hour before storing it. It keeps for up to five days.

Goodbye Oil Shampoo

You will need:

A large bowl used exclusively for shampoo making

Spoon or spatula to mix

Funnel

Jar for storage/bottle

Ingredients:

3 tablespoons of freshly squeezed organic lemon juice

½ cup of organic castile soap

1 teaspoon of organic aloe Vera gel

How to:

Mix together in the bowl until well blended. Place the finished product in the storage container of your choice. This shampoo stays fresh up to five days.

Fight Oil with Oil Shampoo

You will need:
A large bowl used exclusively for shampoo making
Spoon or spatula to mix
Funnel
Jar for storage/bottle

Ingredients:
3 teaspoons of baking soda
1 ripe organic avocado (peeled, pitted and pureed)
¼ cup of warm bottled water (distilled)

How to:
Blend all ingredients in the bowl to form a smooth paste.
Pour the mixture into the storage container. It keeps up to three days.

Oil Be Gone Shampoo

You will need:
A large bowl used exclusively for shampoo making
Spoon or spatula to mix
Funnel
Jar for storage/bottle

Ingredients:

1/3 cup of organic castile soap

¼ cup of organic coconut milk

1 teaspoon of organic almond oil

15 drops of lemon essential oil

5 drops of cinnamon essential oil

How to:

In the bowl, mix the coconut milk and castile soap. Add the almond oil and essential oils. Mix well. Pour the mixture into the storage container. It keeps up to three days. Shake to use.

Our second set of liquid shampoo recipes is for dry hair. Be sure to know very well what type of hair you have, to make the shampoo that will work best for your hair.

Dry hair can be detected by these signs:

- Frizzy hair
- Excessive hair breakage
- Split ends

Any of these signs, or a combination of them, could mean you have dry hair. To better determine your hair type, consult a professional stylist. Use the following recipes as you would shampoo.

Hydration for Thirsty Hair Shampoo

You will need:

A large bowl used exclusively for shampoo making

Spoon or spatula to mix

Funnel

Spray bottle

Ingredients:

1 cup of organic castile soap

¼ cup of water

2 tablespoons of apple cider vinegar

1 tablespoon of tea tree oil

5 drops of jasmine essential oil

How to:

In the bowl, mix all the ingredients together, except the essential oil. Mix well. Pour the mixture into the storage container. Now, add the drops of essential oil on top. Shake well. It keeps up to three days. It is important with this shampoo; that you store it in a spray bottle and shake it well before every use.

Soak in the Moisture Shampoo

You will need:
Food processor
Funnel
Jar/Bottle for storage

Ingredients:
¼ cup of organic castile soap
6 organic garlic cloves (finely chopped)
½ cup of Jojoba oil
1 tablespoon of apple cider vinegar
3 tablespoons of fresh organic apple juice
¼ cup of bottled water (distilled)
5 drops of almond essential oil

How to:
Combine all ingredients in your food processor, on low setting until smooth. Place your shampoo in a storage container. This shampoo can be stored up to seven days.

Moisture Rich Shampoo

You will need:
A large bowl used exclusively for shampoo making

Spoon or spatula to mix

Funnel

Jar/Bottle for storage

Ingredients:

2 teaspoons of olive oil

2 organic eggs

2 teaspoons of lemon juice

3 teaspoons of baking soda

5 drops of lavender essential oil

How to:

In the bowl, beat the two eggs. Add all the other ingredients until the mixture is very smooth. Pour your shampoo into the storage container. This shampoo keeps fresh for no longer than three days.

No More Dryness Shampoo

You will need:

Spoon or spatula to mix

Stovetop pan used exclusively for shampoo making

Funnel

Jar/Bottle for storage

Ingredients:

5 drops of chamomile essential oil

5 drops of carrot seed essential oil

6 tablespoons of bottled water (distilled)

2 tablespoons of raw, organic honey

How to:

In the pan, on low heat, carefully slow melt the honey in the water. The honey should be lightly melted. Stir and remove from heat. Add your essential oils. When fully cool, store your shampoo in a storage container.

Pure Silk Shampoo

You will need:

Spoon or spatula to mix

Funnel

Jar/Bottle for storage

Ingredients:

5 drops of ginger essential oil

2 tablespoons of raw, organic honey

1/4 cup of organic milk

How to:

Mix together honey and milk in a storage container. Add the essential oil drops. Be sure to mix this shampoo before each use. This keeps fresh for two days.

Our third set of liquid shampoo recipes is for normal hair. Be sure to know very well what type of hair you have, to make the shampoo that will work best for your hair.

Normal hair can be detected by these signs:
- Appears healthy
- Not many hair health issues
- Minimal hair loss

Any of these signs, or a combination of them, could mean you have normal hair. To better determine your hair type, consult a professional stylist. Use the following recipes as you would shampoo.

Shine, shine, shine Shampoo

You will need:
A bowl used exclusively for shampoo making
Spoon or spatula to mix
Funnel
Jar/Bottle for storage

Ingredients:
½ cup of bottled water (distilled)
½ cup of organic castile soap
2 tablespoons of almond oil

5 drops of rosemary essential oil

How to:

In the bowl, mix the castile soap and water until blended. Add the almond oil, mix. Let this mixture set for twenty minutes. After it is set, add the essential oil. Pour the shampoo into the storage container. This shampoo keeps well for up to five days.

Bouncy and Silky Shampoo

You will need:
A stovetop pan used exclusively for shampoo making
Spoon or spatula to mix
Funnel
Jar/Bottle for storage

Ingredients:
5 drops of lemon essential oil
1 cup of beer
1 cup of organic castile soap

How to:

Heat the beer up in the pan on low heat, until it is reduced to ¼ a cup. Add the beer to the castile soap, stir well. When cool, add the essential oil. Store shampoo in the storage container. Shampoo keeps well up to seven days.

Aromatic Shine Shampoo

You will need:

A stovetop pan used exclusively for shampoo making

Spoon or spatula to mix

Funnel

Jar/Bottle for storage

Ingredients:

25 drops of ginger essential oil

25 drops of lemon essential oil

25 drops of jasmine essential oil

1/3 cup of canned coconut milk

1/3 cup of organic coconut oil

1 cup of organic castile soap

How to:

Melt together the coconut milk and oil over low heat, stir. It should be lightly melted. Once the mixture is cool, pour the liquid into the storage bottle. Add the castile soap, shake well. Add all the essential oils, shake well again. This will keep up to seven days.

Lively Hair Shampoo

You will need:

A bowl used exclusively for shampoo making

Spoon or spatula to mix

Funnel

Jar/Bottle for storage

Ingredients:

25 drops of orange essential oil

10 drops of lemon essential oil

1/4 cup of organic castile soap

¼ cup of aloe Vera gel

¼ teaspoon of olive oil

How to:

Mix all ingredients EXCEPT the essential oils together in a bowl. When the ingredients are well blended, add your essential oils and mix again. Pour into a storage bottle. Shake this shampoo before every use. It keeps up to seven days.

Radiant Locks Shampoo

You will need:

A bowl used exclusively for shampoo making

Spoon or spatula to mix

Funnel

Jar/Bottle for storage

Ingredients:

25 drops of grapefruit essential oil

¼ cup of bottled water (distilled)

½ teaspoon of sunflower oil

¼ cup of organic castile soap

How to:

Mix the water, soap and sunflower oil together. Once they are well blended, add the essential oil. Put the shampoo in the storage container. This shampoo lasts up to five days.

As you can see, making your own liquid shampoo is easy and fun. They store quite well, just be on the lookout for signs of deterioration. Since you are working with mostly plant base materials, it is best to be careful. It is also important to note that your hair may need a period of adjustment. Using all natural products begins a detoxifying process on your hair. As with anything new we introduce to our body, results are not instantaneous. Be patient, and enjoy your new healthy head of hair.

Chapter 6: Shampoo Bars - For all Hair Types

In this chapter, we will create bar shampoo. The benefits of making your own bar shampoo are that you can make several different kinds. Now, you can have a variety of shampoos at your disposal. Bar shampoo is a multi use; it can be used on the body as well. Just be cautious around the most sensitive area of your genitals. You can purchase natural soaps that are melt and pour, and you won't have to work with lye. Shampoo bars are made in large quantities, but you can cut them and share!

Our first set of shampoo bar recipes will be for dry hair. Be sure to know very well what type of hair you have, to make the shampoo that will work best for your hair. If you are not sure about what type of hair you have, consult your beauty specialist.

Basic to None Shampoo Bar

You will need:
A stove top pan used exclusively for shampoo making
Microwave
Spoon or spatula to mix

Soap molds or bread pan with parchment paper

Rubbing alcohol in spray bottle (fine mist)

Storage container for shampoo bars

Ingredients:

25 drops of grapefruit essential oil

10 drops of ylang ylang essential oil

1 pound of melt and pour organic shea butter soap base

2 tablespoons of olive oil

1 teaspoon of shea butter

How to:

Cut the shea butter base up in cubes, melt the base on *very* low heat, stirring and watching it carefully. When melted turn off but leave in pan. In a microwave safe cup melt the olive oil and shea butter. Add the melted oil and butter to the melted soap base, mix carefully to avoid bubbles. Add the essential oils, again, mixing carefully. Pour the liquid into the mold of your choice. If using a bread pan, make sure the parchment paper overlaps on the sides for easy removal. Be sure that your molds are on a flat surface. Pour bar shampoo mixture into the molds, if bubbles form on the surface once it is poured, spray a bit of rubbing alcohol on top to dissolve them. Let the shampoo bar set overnight, in a cool area. When the shampoo bar is set, gently remove it from the mold. Store your shampoo bar in the storage container. Shampoo bar keeps fresh up to five months, when stored correctly.

Sunny Day Shampoo Bar

You will need:

A stove top pan used exclusively for shampoo making

Microwave

Spoon or spatula to mix

Soap molds or bread pan with parchment paper

Rubbing alcohol in spray bottle (fine mist)

Storage container for shampoo bars

Ingredients:

5 drops of grapefruit essential oil

5 drops of lemon essential oil

1 pound of melt and pour clear organic soap base

1 ½ teaspoons of olive oil

4 teaspoons of shea butter

1 teaspoon almond oil

1 ounce of beeswax

How to:

Cut the soap base up in cubes, melt the base on *very* low heat, stirring and watching it carefully. When melted turn off but leave in pan. In a microwave safe cup melt the oils, (except the essential oils) shea butter, and beeswax. Add the melted oil and butter to the melted soap base, mix carefully to avoid bubbles. Add the essential oils, again, mixing carefully. Pour the liquid into the mold of your choice. If using a bread pan, make sure the parchment paper overlaps on the sides for easy removal. Be sure that your molds are on a flat surface. Pour shampoo bar mixture into the molds, if bubbles form on the surface once it is poured, spray a bit of rubbing alcohol on top to dissolve them. Let the shampoo bar set overnight, in a cool area. When the shampoo bar is set, gently remove it from the mold. Store your shampoo bar in the storage container. Shampoo bars keeps up to five months, if stored correctly.

Our second set of shampoo bar recipes will be for oily hair. Be sure to know very well what type of hair you have, to make the shampoo that will work best for your hair. If you are not sure about what type of hair you have, consult your beauty specialist.

Clean as a Whistle Shampoo Bar

You will need:
A stove top pan used exclusively for shampoo making
Microwave
Spoon or spatula to mix
Soap molds or bread pan with parchment paper

Rubbing alcohol in spray bottle (fine mist)

Storage container for shampoo bars

Ingredients:

15 drops of rosemary essential oil

15 drops of tea tree essential oil

1 pound of melt and pour clear organic soap base

5 teaspoons of Green zeolite clay

How to:

Cut the soap base up in cubes, melt the base on *very* low heat, stirring and watching it carefully. When melted turn off but leave in pan. Add the clay to the melted soap base, mix carefully to avoid bubbles. Add the essential oils, again, mixing carefully. Pour the liquid into the mold of your choice. If using a bread pan, make sure the parchment paper overlaps on the sides for easy removal. Be sure that your molds are on a flat surface. Pour shampoo bar mixture into the molds, if bubbles form on the surface once it is poured, spray a bit of rubbing alcohol on top to dissolve them. Let the shampoo bar set overnight, in a cool area. When the shampoo bar is set, gently remove it from the mold. Store your shampoo bar in the storage container. Shampoo bars keeps up to five months, if stored correctly.

Mother Earth Shampoo Bar

You will need:

A stove top pan used exclusively for shampoo making

Small glass bowl

Spoon or spatula to mix

Soap molds or bread pan with parchment paper

Rubbing alcohol in spray bottle (fine mist)

Storage container for shampoo bars

Ingredients:

1 pound of melt and pour clear organic soap base

1 teaspoon of almond oil

3 drops of rosemary essential oil

7 drops of lavender essential oil

15 drops of orange essential oil

1 drop of clove essential oil

2 teaspoons of ground cinnamon (divided)

How to:

In the small glass bowl, combine all the essential oils and 1 teaspoon of cinnamon. Put aside, but on hand. Cut the soap base up in cubes, melt the base on *very* low heat, stirring and watching it carefully. As it melts, add 1 teaspoon of cinnamon, stirring, but do not over stir. When melted turn off but leave in pan. Immediately add the almond oil and the essential oils blend. Pour the liquid into the mold of your choice. If using a bread pan, make sure the parchment paper overlaps on the sides for easy removal. Be sure that your molds are on a flat surface. Pour shampoo bar mixture into the molds, if bubbles form on the surface once it is poured, spray a bit of rubbing alcohol on top to dissolve them. Let the shampoo bar set overnight, in a cool area. When the shampoo bar is set, gently remove it from the mold. Store your shampoo bar in the storage container. Shampoo bars keeps up to five months, if stored correctly.

Our third set of shampoo bar recipes will be for normal hair. Be sure to know very well what type of hair you have, to make the shampoo that will work best for your hair. If you are not sure about what type of hair you have, consult your beauty specialist.

True Shine Shampoo Bar

You will need:
A stove top pan used exclusively for shampoo making
Small glass bowl
Spoon or spatula to mix
Soap molds or bread pan with parchment paper
Rubbing alcohol in spray bottle (fine mist)
Storage container for shampoo bars

Ingredients:

2 pounds of melt and pour clear organic soap base

10 drops of chocolate essential oil

1/2 teaspoon of cocoa butter

½ mango butter

1 teaspoon of almond oil

How to:

Cut the soap base up in cubes, melt the base with the butter on *very* low heat, stirring and watching it carefully. When melted, turn off but leave in pan. Immediately add the almond oil and the essential oils blend. Pour the liquid into the mold of your choice. If using a bread pan, make sure the parchment paper overlaps on the sides for easy removal. Be sure that your molds are on a flat surface. Pour shampoo bar mixture into the molds, if bubbles form on the surface once it is poured, spray a bit of rubbing alcohol on top to dissolve them. Let the shampoo bar set overnight, in a cool area. When the shampoo bar is set, gently remove it from the mold. Store your shampoo bar in the storage container. Shampoo bars keeps up to five months, if it is stored correctly.

Sweet Smell Shampoo Bar

You will need:

A stove top pan used exclusively for shampoo making

Small glass bowl

Spoon or spatula to mix

Soap molds or bread pan with parchment paper

Rubbing alcohol in spray bottle (fine mist)

Storage container for shampoo bars

Ingredients:

2 pounds of melt and pour clear organic soap base

4 teaspoons of dried rosemary leaves

15 drops of lemon essential oil

15 drops of lime essential oil

How to:

Cut the soap base up in cubes, melt the base with the butter on *very* low heat, stirring and watching it carefully. When melted, turn off but leave in pan. Add the oils and mix well, but do not over stir. Pour the liquid into the mold of your choice. If using a bread pan, make sure the parchment paper overlaps on the sides for easy removal. Be sure that your molds are on a flat surface. Pour shampoo bar mixture into the molds, if bubbles form on the surface once it is poured, spray a bit of rubbing alcohol on top to dissolve them. Let the shampoo bar set overnight, in a cool area. When the shampoo bar is set, gently remove it from the mold. Store your shampoo bar in the storage container. Shampoo bars keeps up to five months, if stored correctly.

Shampoo bars are useful, last long and cost effective. When stored properly, they can be wonderful for travel. Just cut them up and you're on your way.

Chapter 7: Dry Shampoo - For all Hair Types

Dry shampoos are useful when you don't have as much time as you'd like to wash your hair. They can eliminate odors; give your hair volume and shine. They are great to have on hand when traveling. They can be used while you're camping, when there may not be showers readily accessible. They save both time and money. Dry shampoos are not so hair type specific as they are function specific. The following recipes can be used for all types of hair, find one that works best for you, and make a big batch!

Cornstarch Hair Magic

Just add a bit of cornstarch to the roots of a dry hair. Blend it thoroughly, and then brush it out. That's it, simple. You can store some in a pretty jar in your bathroom or in a container for on the go use.

Baking Soda and Oatmeal Hair Wonder

Combine one cup of finely ground oatmeal with one cup of baking soda. Put it on the roots of your hair, work it in, and then brush it out. Store in a jar for those days when you just don't feel like wet shampooing.

Flour Power Hair

Choose any flour, but consider white flour for light hair, oat flour for dark hair. Work some into the roots of your hair, and then brush it out. This gives extra volume to your hair as well. Store it in a jar to have on hand for those "lazy" days.

Tips for dry shampoos:
You can scent your dry shampoos with dried herbs and flowers, just be sure they are finely ground.
All dry shampoos have up to a month storage period.
Dry shampoos are a great gift at slumber parties and camp gatherings.

Conclusion

In conclusion, these recipes will help you to create your personal hair hygiene. Through testing the recipes, you will discover the joy of making your own products, at a fraction of the cost. Meanwhile, you are veering away from harmful products and practices.

The best way for an ecologically mindful person is to control what you consume. Mindfully abstaining from putting a chemical cocktail on your hair helps it to restore its natural beauty. That is what everyone is seeking, to have beautiful hair that represents our love for mother earth.

www.ingramcontent.com/pod-product-compliance
Lightning Source LLC
Chambersburg PA
CBHW071300280526
45788CB00004B/1786